Becoming Un-Twined

6 Steps to Finding "Me" And Keeping "WE"

Cyndi Rutherford

Dedication

I dedicate this book to you, Bruce, my husband of 5 years, who, when needed, has been strong for me when I was weak. You have encouraged me at the times when writing this book was difficult and being a younger twin yourself, you understand me profoundly. *Iron Sharpens Iron*...we have been told we are a great couple, and I think this is because we support and love each other in so many ways, strengthening our bonds of love.

I also dedicate this book to my three amazing children, Carrie Lynn, Paul Jan, and Christopher Joseph.

Carrie, my oldest, married to Vincent, together they have 4 beautiful boyz, ages 2-12. You have blossomed into a woman who I am so grateful to be your Mom. You are an extremely accomplished woman, who after serving in the United States Army, now has your Masters' degree in engineering. One reason I am so proud of you is that your work ethic and principles are your guiding light. You are a passionate, loving wife and mother, daughter and sister.

My oldest and beloved son Paul, is a reminder that our children are gifts from God to love and nurture, and they are loaned to us for a time unknown to us. Paul, you were only here for 25 short years, but in those years, you lived a lifetime. You have left an indelible impact on those who knew you. You are the most passionate person I knew, and staunch in your personal beliefs and principles. Your heart had an amazing capacity for joy and love. You are incredibly missed and loved.

And to my youngest son, Christopher, who I call "my angel". You saved my life when I was diagnosed with pre-cancer during my pregnancy. You are truly an amazing man. He is married to his wife Andie, they have twins, another daughter, and another son on the way. I am so proud to be your Mom watching you grow into a "gentle giant." You also have a great capacity for love. Your heart is as wide and deep as the ocean, and you seem to have an eternal spring of light within you.

I also want to dedicate this book to my twin, Gail, who has helped me transform in ways which were beyond anything I could conceive.

Last but not least, I dedicate this book to the God of my understanding, Jesus, my Savior, who saved me from myself, who lifted me up out of the ashes to new heights, who put a dream in my heart, and helps me daily to become the woman I am co-creating to be.

Acknowledgements and Thank You

It has been my experience that writing my first book does not happen without the help and support of brilliant creators who are really servants at heart.

I would like to thank Dr. Angela Lauria, the creator of The Author Incubator for her genius in developing a protocol and program which helped me craft, create and execute my first book. I would like to further thank her wonderful, staff who worked closely with me as my developing editor, Ora North, my managing editor, Cory Hott, and my final editor, Madeline Kosten, who altogether were an incredible team bringing their collective talents for inspiration, wisdom, and persistence, and therefore, my book was created.

I would also like to acknowledge and thank The Health Coach Institute, and co-founders Stacy Morgenstern and Carey Peters, for developing a brilliant program and co-creating along with the Success Coaches, TCM© Coaches, and Master Mind Coaches where I am currently enrolled for Holistic Mastery certification. They are my amazing mentors who have had an incredible and amazing impact on my journey toward making a difference for others.

Both of these entities, The Author Incubator, and The Health Coach Institute have coached me, mentored me, and enabled me in my own personal journey to widen my capacity to truly make a difference in the world.

Table of Contents

Chapter 1

Identity Crisis – Was It a "Breakdown" or a "Breakthrough?"

"Life's wisdom comes through the ups and downs."

Although I did not know it, a real problem I was having in my life was that I needed to become who I was apart from my twin, or I would continue to lack independence and a life of my own. This dependency went on for many years, and I struggled with many conflicting thoughts and feelings, as I tried to identify what was wrong with me.

I seemed to be invisible in my relationship with my twin. While she seemed to have found a normal life, I was unable to, and the reason behind this was beyond me. I was so frustrated because it seemed that I was always compromising myself in order to have peace in my relationship with my twin. I struggled with not feeling good enough, and no matter how much I tried to please my twin, I never felt worthy. Although I tried to change my twin, that didn't work. There seemed to be an enormous gap in our relationship, and I just didn't know how to fix it!

I felt like my hands were tied, and although my twin didn't speak to me, I still could not figure out why. I blamed her, she blamed me, and we were just stuck, never connecting on common ground. Yes, there was an enormous gap: how could I find my own identity and be true to myself, while still having my twin?

Since this was my first experience being a twin, I had no clue what a healthy twin relationship should resemble. I had formed my own ideas of what our relationship should look like and based on our parents' – and the world's – expectations of being a twin, I formed my own opinions.

Here are the ideals, expectations, and misconceptions which I perceived to be true: my twin and I were supposed to be very close, we were supposed to share everything and be happy about it, we were supposed to dress alike and like the same style. In addition, we were supposed to have the same friends, and we were never supposed to fight. As a teen, I became aware that none of this was true. I felt very conflicted about what a twin's identity and relationship should be, and I felt significantly conflicted when people would ask me if we were close, because I did not know the answer to that question.

I was the younger twin by only five minutes, but you would think my twin was much older than me. She was the dominant caretaker and I was the passive, dependent, and sensitive twin. I was very vulnerable to criticism and would take things to heart very easily, so I ended up being hurt often.

On the other hand, my twin seemed to roll with the punches and be resilient, while it took me a long time to get the same resilience. Looking back, I am sure I was a real pain to my twin at times. When we were only eight years old, our mother became quite ill and debilitated from brain tumor surgery, and as she needed significant care herself, it was very challenging for her to be nurturing to us. Having this huge void in our lives only accentuated the unhealthy relationship between me and my twin.

In some ways, our relationship was a blessing and a curse. We formed a tight bond and started caring for each other. As my sister was older, although I wasn't conscious of it at the time, she became a mother figure to me. I was a child and I needed my mom, and I didn't realize how this immense expectation was affecting our twin-ship. Being the over dependent twin, I expected much from my sister and when she couldn't deliver, I felt very disappointed, as if she just wasn't there for me. On the other side of that coin, because my sister was the caretaker, she needed to be supported as well. As I was the dependent/passive twin, I was not able to provide this support, and I'm sure my sister felt the same feeling of disappointment.

As my twin filled the role of dominant/caretaking twin, I felt like she was always telling me what to do, and we would get into a lot of fights. With twins, fighting is inevitable, because it is a way of establishing that we are *not* the same person, as the many misconceptions about twins are telling us. We went to parochial grammar school and wore uniforms, so there wasn't individuality for anyone at school. I saw no differences between people. When we entered high school and we were allowed to choose what we wore, I started to see that I was not my twin. In fact, we had very different tastes. Oh boy, did this ever rock the boat! In our household, more fighting began. Because we were being raised to believe the misconceptions about what it means to be a twin, the level and intensity of our fighting only increased.

For me, the real conflict surrounded the fact that I seemed to have a love/hate relationship with having my own independence yet feeling so dependent on my twin. My sister's caretaking enabled and reinforced this passive/dependent role for me. Sometimes our emotions would be so intense, we would need a cooling off period, and we did not know how to contain our emotions in a way that would maintain a close attachment.

When I was younger, I didn't have the awareness I gratefully have today, and I carried a lot of guilt and shame because I felt that I was "bad." Much later in life, I was able to realize that within this struggle was a pathway to gaining my own autonomy, and I wanted my twin to be happy at the same time. I wanted to find my own competency and my own identity apart from my twin.

It is typical for twins to have a strong attachment to each other – one which knew no bounds. "Healthy boundaries" was not a term I was aware of, and it was not something which we practiced. We were so emotionally intertwined that I couldn't see where one of us started and the other ended – this is called *enmeshment*. I could remember an incident when we were five-years-old in school. The blackboard kept repeatedly falling on my sister's head, and I remember feeling so embarrassed for her. Although my twin seemed to be okay with the experience, my emotions did not. I felt so much devotion to her.

It is natural for twins to always be compared – at least, we always were. We were compared physically, academically, and socially, as there are certain expectations for twins which are higher than the expectations for siblings. It is easy to understand but is it not in twins' best interest. This may sound a little crazy to non-twins, but twins will understand this. Comparisons start in early childhood and are adopted by the child as we model our parents. I felt I was either better than or less than my twin, and this did not result in a balanced relationship. In fact, making these comparisons and setting up unrealistic expectations was not helpful in building my self-esteem. I continued to feel like I could never measure up to my twin.

I did not want to participate in situations in which my twin would not engage, because it would feel like I was cheating on her, and I felt like I was being disloyal in some way, threatening the closeness of our twin-ship. For example, we both started to date at the same time, and we dated best friends. I did not consider whether or not I was truly ready to date, I just followed what my twin did. My twin was married before I was, so I knew that at 20-years-old, I needed to start looking for a husband. If I did not, I would feel behind, and I wasn't having any of that.

If these twin issues weren't enough, there were other, bigger problems lurking beneath the surface that began to be revealed.

At the age of 17, my mother died from her long-standing, ten-year illness – we were motherless at such a young age. Three short years later, I married at the age of 20 and moved away due to my husband's job. I left everything behind: my twin, family, my friends – all while I was grieving the loss of my mother. The separation from everything was too much for me and there was a huge void in my life. I began to use alcohol to fill this emptiness and to help me forget everything causing me pain.

Then came my breakdown. and life had abruptly stopped for me. It was gut-wrenching, and painful, and necessary for me to take a break. It was time for me to just *stop*! I was in the midst of a crisis – my *identity crisis*. I did not know who I was at all.

I asked myself, "Who am I?" Still, I did not know the answer. I knew I had roles in life that I played, I knew the color of my hair and eyes, but I did not know what I wanted for myself. I spent most of my life in comparing myself with my twin, living in reaction to others, and not making any deliberate choices for myself. I lived to please others, because I felt so "less than," and invisible, and believed that what I wanted really didn't matter. My upbringing and these experiences led me to a place where I became suicidal, but I had three beautiful children, and they helped me to hang on for one more day – until one day turned into another, and another. This was an opportunity, a blessing in disguise for me to have a new start in life.

As I looked back, what felt like a breakdown was really my breakthrough. Life in all its grace and goodness was offering me a *choice*, and this *choice* is what made the *difference*. I could have stayed afraid and remained stuck in my life, having a really miserable existence, lacking direction and purpose. I had no joy, no love, and no peace. Emotionally, I was experiencing depression, low energy, ambivalence, uncertainty, loneliness, and anxiety. All of this was affecting my relationship with my twin, my family and friends and co-workers.

Staying in my familiar place was very tempting, but I needed to consider the cost. Defending my ego would be deadly. Was this worth it? As risky as it felt, I knew in my gut I could not go back to the way I had been living. As risky as it felt, I had to move forward; what was ahead couldn't possibly be any worse. My life change amounted to taking a leap of faith into the unknown, which felt so foreign to me, having not experienced it until that moment. Taking the risk, I lived to become spiritually sober first, and then I was able to find my identity. I was given the opportunity and freedom to let go of what wasn't serving me. This offered me the opportunity to start on the journey of discovering my identity apart from my twin, and you can have the same experience!

What happens when you start on a journey of discovering your own identity? You will begin to unravel your feelings, your misconceptions, and expectations others have had for you, and you get to *decide*. You will begin to own and appreciate everything about yourself – your thoughts, feelings, personality, and your own DNA. You will sense a new freedom and happiness, and you will start to really live in a new way being comfortable in your own skin. Your feelings and your perceptions change by being open, trusting and believing in yourself. It starts a revolution in the universe for positive opportunities and outcomes to come to you. You will experience more alignment with a Power Greater, and your life will become amazing, instead of miserable because of all these things that were put upon you. You *get to decide what you want.* That's *freedom.*

What I have described for you here is an anatomy of some of the dilemmas you experience as a twin, based on my own experiences. These describe my "younger twin self," and not who I am today.

Although this book provides many moments for self-reflection, it also provides a process for healing from the issues of your own twin-ship. You have a decision to maintain the status quo, or to move forward towards having your own true identity, living an independent life apart from your twin, while still having your twin in your life.

Chapter 2

The Faulty Foundation –

Collapsing the "Old Story"

"Release the pressure to create change and focus on increasing choice."

Were you given the same wisdom with very little choice? I was told to "play well the cards life deals you." I do not hear choice in this "wisdom." This was the wisdom of the times. Or I heard, "you made your bed, now lie in it." This sounds like what I call "stuck-ness," and there doesn't seem to be much choice in the matter! This was some of the beginnings of my programming and being the passive/compliant twin, I accepted this sort of philosophy, no questions asked, as dark as it seems.

You may or may not relate, but you were definitely given an "old story." So, what do I mean by that? These ideas and beliefs are faulty foundations, and I think it's important to give you some background on who I will call my "younger twin" and her experience growing up as a child, filled with so much pain, trauma, and disappointment.

My life didn't start out this way. It started with hope and promise, but our mother suddenly had a brain tumor leading to surgery at age 39 and was left paralyzed on her left side. At only eight years old, our lives flipped upside down. I became the caretaker for my mom – or, as much of a caretaker as I could be at that age. My childhood as I knew it – happy and fun – was now sad and hard. My childhood was gone, and this was coupled with our father's drinking in order to cope with his disappointment. Because of the stress in our household there was an enormous strain on our family, and the foundation of my life with my twin was built upon pain, sadness and disappointment – add to this the faulty foundation of misconceptions, expectations, comparisons, and codependency. I called our home the "house of pain," and I learned how to "stuff" my feelings; there was no place to put them, so my feelings were repressed. I thought I had tucked them neatly away forever, but they started coming out sideways in strange ways, evident in my inappropriate behavior and misplaced anger.

As far as having our parents being present, my twin and I were motherless and fatherless. With both of our parents being ill in different ways, we appeared to be growing up fast, but this was just an illusion – I wasn't growing up at all. Instead, this was simply how we learned to survive. I learned how to escape, and I started looking for love in all the wrong places, trying to get the love and nurturing that I was missing.

My grandmother was my "rock star." She took care of all our basic needs, and she provided emotional comfort and support along with taking care of our physical needs. She showed me the way of faith and prayer, although I was not ready to embark on a spiritual path yet. She was my angel; a stable presence in the midst of chaos and heartache and who I loved to be near.

My Messages

I learned that life was disappointing and unreliable, and that your world could be shattered in a moment's notice, just like that! As I was growing up, I was not consciously aware that I was forming these beliefs. The messages I was getting and internalizing were that everyone would disappoint me sooner or later, and there was no one I could rely on or trust to be there for me. I became distant and I isolated myself from people. I became self-sufficient, and I felt deeply disappointed and let down by my parents, life, and God. I started making my own decisions – the good, the bad, and the ugly. I felt as if I didn't need anyone; after all, no one was ever there for me.

I had to start taking care of myself. There was so much anger and resentment brewing in me, that I just wanted to retaliate for all the hurt and pain that was inside me. However, I kept it hidden inside, starting to live a double life as a teen, keeping in all these secrets with so much shame.

As I looked around, I didn't see any evidence of family that came close to resembling mine. I felt so abnormal and I pretended I was happy. Who in the world had time to listen anyway? People were busy living their lives. I felt so conflicted. I became an actress – not a paid actress, but I was an expert at pretending. As long I looked good on the outside, no one would know how I was feeling. This was my plan! I would just act the part. If my face would slip, I would just keep applying that make-up so no one could see inside me, and I put on a smile as best I could. I wore this facade for many years that it became one of my survival tools. Academically, I made it through high school with average grades. Our mother was dying in our senior year, and I was so depressed that I missed the last ten days of school – I just couldn't show up anymore. After all, what was the point? There would be no one showing up for our graduation. I was painfully empty. When our graduation rolled around, my twin and I were there by ourselves, just another day in our lives. I remember feeling so embarrassed, just sticking out like a sore thumb, which everyone could see.

Our mom died right after our graduation on September 20th of that year, and I felt like a contestant on the show *Naked and Afraid*. I learned that I could escape into alcohol and it would fix the way I felt inside – at least temporarily.

I spent the next ten years trying diligently to bury the pain I felt, because it was too painful to feel. That ride came to an end when alcohol was no longer working. I saw myself becoming something I did not want to be. It was time for a change, and I needed help. I wanted something better for my children than what I had growing up.

At 33-years-old, as I mentioned in the previous chapter, my insides were falling apart – surprise, surprise! In hindsight, it was probably the best experience for me. It felt like all the faulty foundation inside me was crumbing and collapsing, and I could see a thousand pieces of glass breaking and falling to the ground. That, was the "old story" shattering inside me. I felt completely untethered to everything I once held dear – everything that was familiar.

Something had happened to me, but was it a *breakdown* or a *breakthrough*? I saw this as my opportunity to change my life.

Do you want to have breakthrough? Although your transformation doesn't need to be as dramatic as mine, you too can collapse your "old story," and break free of your old "stuff," creating a new identity more in alignment with who you are.

This breakthrough begins with building a new awareness of what you want for yourself.

You are not a mistake; you are not being punished. You can grow past your faulty foundation which was a part of your development, clearing this away so you can begin to artfully carve and create who you are – your own identity – being a stand-alone person next to your twin, without being enmeshed.

The strong attachment my twin and I had early on was complicated by issues of co-dependency and addiction. Because of these issues, I had challenges when I tried to develop a healthy sense of self.

The mystique of being a twin gets installed when we are still in the womb. The misconceptions and expectations that are put on twins is just craziness as far as I'm concerned, but I understand it is inevitable. Still, this causes conflicts and self-doubt in the twin-ship. While it was fun for me to always have a playmate, my twin was labeled the dominant twin, and as she started making friends outside our twin-ship, I became labeled the shy, quiet twin, and felt alone. I was not as socially adaptable as my twin sister.

By understanding your past and gaining a new perspective, you will have a greater sense of yourself and a more authentic relationship with your twin. Developing self-awareness of your own identity as an individual, and as a twin, is a very special and worthwhile process. Unpacking the twin mystique is a very difficult experience and sometimes causes struggles in the twin relationship. Up until I understood this, I felt *alone* with such thoughts as, "Twins who are close, don't fight." This certainly fit nicely into the concept of the twin mystique, and I carried a secret of shame because of it. Knowing there are normal upsides and downsides is freeing, because I wanted to keep this secret belief and unhappiness to myself. It is hard to get others to understand the nature of this pain when you are misunderstood, ignored, or perceived as being dramatic or overly sensitive.

People say, "Once a twin, always a twin." Although fighting can become a strategy in trying to become an individual, this doesn't work very well. If the fighting continues, there is a danger of becoming estranged from your twin, and how sad and lonely is that? Accepting there will be times when you and your twin are not going to see eye-to-eye is important. As I have grown, I have been freed from forcing similarities between us, and have grown to accept our differences, and to live and let live. We will not always share the same opinion, thoughts, or feelings, and that is just a part of having your own identity. It is not a *sin*. You are not your twin – you are who you are and finding yourself apart from your twin can be the most exciting, freeing, and happy new journey. You can give yourself the freedom to be yourself, so pack a suitcase with all the essentials and take the trip! You will forever be happy and grateful you decided this, and you will have a deeper connection with yourself and your twin.

I had to collapse the "old story" of unworthiness, feeling not good enough and invisibility. I also needed to come to terms with the hidden false beliefs, and embrace the idea of being self-sufficient - that I could change what I hadn't been able to change on my own before. By letting go of the victim mentality I could stop asking myself questions like, "Why is my twin doing this to me?" I was blaming my twin. This was the result of having a victim mentality which bred irresponsibility for my own choices. And this kind of negative thinking kept me stuck in my "old story."

Like Dorothy in *"The Wizard of Oz,"* you will see you always had the power to go home, you just didn't realize it" you become free to choose your own happiness. No one is responsible for your happiness, and no one can withhold your happiness….the power is within you and isn't that great news?

You do not have to be beholden or in bondage to one another; you hold the keys to your Kingdom of Happiness, and this truly calls for a celebration. Having your own identity apart from your twin and being free from all that held you back from having the life you dream of, while still having your twin in your life, is quite an accomplishment!

I've written this chapter with a dual purpose in mind. I want you to know that I have been where you are, my friend, and I want to help you build the awareness of your programming, as well as your faulty foundation, and how this impacts you, your twin-ship, and other relationships. You may have felt like you were crazy at times – fighting with your twin caused resentment, frustration, and dis-ease. You may have felt so conflicted, as you did not have any clear sense of who you were apart from your twin, living with happiness so far out of your reach, and bucking under the pressure of all those expectations! All this pressure to be someone you are not, doing things you feel you should in order to please others, feeling disoriented and pulled in many directions, without clear boundaries, and not being aligned with who you uniquely are – this is a recipe for disaster! Boundaries are so important to guarantee stability in your life – they keep you in your lane, so you can enjoy real peace of mind. Boundaries are an indication of your own self-respect and values which guide your decisions and keep you growing.

Transforming co-dependency to God-dependency (or insert the name of your higher power here) will catapult you into a completely different dimension of your life – it's like trading in an old beat up vehicle for a brand-new shiny one.

I would have given anything to have had the *road map* I've laid out in the next chapter.

What would you do to have your dream come true?

Chapter 3

Follow the Yellow Brick Road –

It Leads to Your Heart

"Without a Vision, the People Perish"

You may say, "A vision? Really? Where do I even begin?"

I believe any new beginning starts with *desire*! Most people believe transformation starts with a mindset and behavior change, and although these are vital aspects to change, you are entitled to so much more – you are entitled to a real, lasting, and deep change that begins in your heart. Your heart is the container which holds your deepest desires. What is in your "heart of hearts?" What is it that makes you feel *alive*? What is it that has you feel a *fire* in your soul?

As you dive into this chapter, you will understand that you have a clear path to co-create your unique vision and an opportunity to paint a portrait of your unique life as an individual, based on what it is that is important to *only you*!

You will also understand that as you connect with your vision, you will have a measurable process to break through your "stuckness," and discover what is holding you back from the life you deserve to have.

This is a process of moving you from "stuck" to having *choice*!

What does this process require? It takes *making a decision* and a *commitment to yourself*!

The most significant reason I could not move forward in my life I was *stuck*! For me, "stuckness" was not knowing I had a choice – that was just the way it was. Remember, the programming I received, "the cards life dealt me?" I just accepted this as my reality! I didn't know there was a banquet in the next room, because what held me back were limiting beliefs I owned. I told myself I did not deserve more, and on the heels of this belief was the thought that , "it is selfish to want more – just be content with what you have." There was no road map or a design for living – at least, not one that I was aware of. As a result, I was settling in life, but there was a Power Greater than I who wanted to give me so much more. I was standing in my own way, but I did not know it. Another limiting belief is that God is a reluctant God!

These limiting beliefs have to go, and this is what I want for you, my friend – to dream and to *dream big*!

One of the most common spots to be stuck in, is *indecision*! There are many reasons why obstacles can occur for you, such as having your priorities mixed up, or wanting to please everyone but yourself. Although it feels conflicting, you must consider your own needs so as not to neglect yourself. I believe codependents have difficulty making decisions because they become so absorbed in taking care of others people's problems, they don't have time to identify or solve their own issues. Codependents feel so responsible for others because the people around them care so little, so they are always picking up the slack, leading to resentment towards the other person. On the other hand, codependents have to fix everything, so they feel responsible to hold it all together. That's a lot of pressure to deal with daily.

Another reason it may be difficult to make decisions is because you are in *reaction* to everyone and everything around you. You may be reacting to all your thoughts, feelings, behaviors, as well as everyone else's thoughts, feelings, opinions, and problems. Now, reacting is a part of being alive and being a human being, but when it can be described as overly reactive, or when it gets to a point where you are upset almost every day, making mistakes and creating stress – this is where your reactive state has gone too far. It is difficult to make decisions when you are being tossed about like a leaf in the wind in every direction being "ungrounded." Living in this unstable condition; your emotions are actually being controlled by "outside" interference.

Living in a state of continual turmoil makes it extremely difficult for you to focus on yourself.

Remember, I said earlier, "Real transformation happens within your heart."

Living in a more grounded space, you are reflective, thoughtful, and intuitive, and you have a more introspective view living your life from the inside out, and not from the outside in. Living this way will allow you to be better in tune and aligned with who you are, and will enable you to make much better choices. This way, you will have greater clarity and peace for yourself, and for your loved ones.

"The journey of 1000 steps begins with the first step," so making a decision and closely connecting to this decision builds your commitment. Your result/outcome will be based on how well you have formed your goal, which I will discuss in more detail in a later chapter. It will depend on how well you trust the process, how much you want something better for yourself, and how deserving you believe you are to have what you want.

While we are hanging out here, discussing making a decision, I think it is also wise to see what happens if you try to change on your own effort alone, or if you choose to just read this book and put the lessons within these pages aside for another time. I have tried the strategy of doing it myself, because I simply just thought I could. I did not know any better. Hey, nothing ventured, nothing gained, right? It's okay – there is no failure, only feedback, and the feedback I received was that doing it myself did not work very well. I would procrastinate; I would not follow through; I would give myself all kinds of excuses and they all sounded good to me! I was missing the opportunity to build momentum by not working with someone who cared enough to hold me accountable to my desired state. Growth doesn't happen in isolation; it happens in community with others, so I needed to become willing to come out of my comfort zone and be uncomfortable for a little while. The good news is that "this too shall pass" – nothing is permanent, and everything is in flow. I needed people to either kick me in the butt when I needed it, or to love me enough to be honest with me when I was going backwards, helping me to stay true to my ideal, desired state. Making a decision to follow through will expand your growth exponentially and stretch you to be in greater alignment with yourself.

Okay, so let's say you read this book and decide you want to disregard it. I feel compelled to speak the truth, and say, "Nothing Changes if Nothing Changes," because it is true. Perhaps you are not ready for this journey. What will it take for you to be ready? What are you feeling over and over, and how are your feelings affecting your mood/motivation in your daily life? Are you feeling a great deal of frustration because you wish something would change, but it does not? Wishing is only for children blowing out candles on their birthday cake. Is this still working for you? Or, like me, are you giving yourself a set of excuses, but not realizing that you are. Or, even worse, are you aware that you are giving yourself these excuses, and have given up and quit on yourself? If this is you, just making one choice will begin the process of transformation.

The road map for transforming your "old story" into creating a "new story" is built on a firm foundation and is laid out in six steps:

1. Stepping Back
2. Letting Go
3. Exploring and Connecting to Spirituality
4. Co-Creating the "Real" You from Your Heart's Desire
5. Forgiveness
6. Taking Empowered Action: Saying Yes to Yourself

The steps in this process are purposefully designed to be taken in this order. This is your process and it is unique to you – it is not cookie cutter or "one size fits all" here. So you can move through at your own pace. The steps are meant to fulfill the desires of your heart – to build your own unique identity, help you know who you truly are, and they are designed to help you to co-create your unique identity, while learning how to navigate a complicated twin relationship and still be true to yourself.

Have you ever really taken the time to step back from your life to get a different perspective? Please consider that I do not recommend you do it the way I did years ago, resulting in a nervous breakdown, so give yourself a long overdue break. But if you do have a breakdown, that's okay too. I hold no regrets after my episode, and I accept my life as being exactly as it was supposed to be – this was a gift sent to me by the Spirit of the Universe and it was a time for me to receive feedback. It was a time for listening. It was a time for being still, trusting, and letting go – for surrendering to a Power Greater than me.

Step One: Stepping Back

When you are in the midst of a problem, we become so focused on the problem we cannot see the possibility of having a new resource or solution. The purpose of stepping back is to create more possibility and more choice. It is like looking through a different set of lenses. Stepping back and creating distance from you and your programming gives you the opportunity to have a change in your perspective. This is a very powerful concept. Stepping back and looking out as an observer frees you from your emotional reaction to the situation, and opens you up to a calm state, creating a different view.

Step Two: Letting Go

Letting go is a very powerful tool. The purpose here is to unhinge the "old beliefs," which are creating the same repetitive experience for you, and contributing to your present state. If you didn't need this step in your life, you would not be reading this book. Because of childhood programming, patterns of behavior and predictable thinking – it is like being in a black and white movie, without color or vibrancy. Things are boring and generate low energy. This step takes courage, because this is where fear conspires to convince you not to let go – fear of the unknown could stop you in your tracks, or it will cause you to second guess yourself. If you let them, fear and doubt will discourage you from moving forward and reaching your desired state.

Step Three: Exploring and Connecting to Spirituality

Choosing a spiritual path is a totally unique and individual journey. There are many ways which lead to a Power Greater, and you have the opportunity to choose a concept of your own understanding. I believe that learning to live in greater alignment and purpose is an invitation open to all.

Step Four: Co-Creating the "Real" You from Your Heart's Desire

This step is all about creating who you've always wanted to be. However, now you will recognize just what has been holding you back from finding your voice, your own competency without being under the control of your twin, and your own truth, and it is about stepping into and being comfortable in your own skin, emerging as your true self, letting go of your "false self," and growing into a new dimension of your life.

Step Five: Forgiveness

The fifth step is vital to your growth and healing. It is all about forgiving yourself for not knowing, and forgiving others for not knowing. This is the step which will free you from the emotional baggage you've been carrying. Now you can "drop the rock," releasing hurts from your past, both those you caused and those done unto you.

You're almost there! Thanks for hanging in there; you're doing great!

Step Six: Taking Empowered Action

In other words, this step is about saying yes to yourself! You are re-claiming yourself through taking desired action and being accountable to yourself because you are worth more than your weight in gold! Without taking the desired action, there is no forward movement, no momentum to build toward what you want, and staying true to your core values. If your forgiveness is not received, you will still grow, because you have forgiven. This is really a matter of the heart.

When you are saying *no* to yourself, have you thought about what you are saying *yes* to? This is a "blind spot" for many called denial.

This is the principle of cause and effect. For example, if your goal is to lose ten pounds, you've just said *no* to that chocolate cake, and you've said *yes* to your desires to lose those ten pounds. How are you feeling? Are you empowered, and happy to do that again? Let your answer be yes! Each time you say *no* to your present state of being overweight by ten pounds, you are saying *yes* to your desired state of having what you want.

It's always wise to look at the other side of that coin. Imagine saying no to yourself – you are really saying no to what you want, or your desired state. You have now shifted yourself out of alignment, and you are getting more of what you don't want.

Uh--oh! What happens next? Everything shifts with that – feelings of disempowerment and disappointment enter, or maybe you even beat yourself up, leading to that same old sad song again, "I'm a failure." Your "old programming" begins to rear its ugly head.

Saying *yes* to yourself in ways that bring more alignment with your true self brings you assurance, confidence, empowerment, and success.

So, here's to your *success*!

Chapter 4

Seeing Through A New Lens

"Everything is possible, and there is always a way."

You cannot build a structure until you first envision it, develop a blueprint, and begin to structure it. The same is true for your life. This first steps in this process is in two parts, 1. stepping back and 2. letting go. It will lead you to uncovering obstacles which have kept you stuck, recognizing patterns of thought and behavior – attributing to feeling victimized – and opening to the idea that it may be the right time to let go of your inner "younger twin."

I prided myself on being a super responsible person – I was self-sufficient, independent, and I could handle anything that came my way. But this could not be further from the truth.

The truth was, my life was very unmanageable, but no one could tell me that. I just thought that if everyone would just behave themselves my "world" would be okay. I did not know it at the time, but I was completely closed to something new or different because I was convinced that my way was *the* way. I was completely – no doubts whatsoever – convinced that all the answers were in my head. After all, I was a fairly intellectual person, I could reason things out into various outcomes, but I was not getting the outcomes I wanted. One of the reasons I was not having positive outcomes, very simply, was that I did not know what I wanted. A part of me wanted to find myself and be free and a part of me wanted to play it safe and stay the same (no changing). Life was beginning to grab my attention.

I would often find myself in a state of feeling confused, upset, distraught, at the end of my rope, overwhelmed, angry, frustrated or filled with despair, and collapse. I had a whole lot of self-directed will. And so, what would I do? You guessed it! I would redouble my efforts at control. I would try harder and I would do better and be better, because I never felt good enough – my programming was at work again! I would repeat this pattern of thought and behavior from the programming I received as a child. This just came naturally to me. It was what I knew – it was familiar to me. I did not know what I did not know.

I have to just take a moment to say that I have completely forgiven both my parents. They provided the best they could under the most difficult circumstances, and

I want you to know that you can have this same peace with your past.

When I would come from a place of self-directed will, for example, I would try to force solutions, driven by all the emotions I mentioned earlier. The main culprits were fear and anger. These two emotions were my constant companions, and my thinking became quite distorted. So, my go-to place was to go into my head and wallow in my familiar framework. I was not open to a Power Greater than myself or my own heart or intuition because I filled was with so much self-doubt and distrust.

Needless to say, I was not getting the outcomes I wanted as a result. Instead, I was having a lot of stress and tension in my relationship with my twin. I practiced distancing myself until the present situation would just be forgotten. But was it really forgotten? The answer is no! I was burying my feelings in order to avoid conflict. Remember, I mentioned I was the passive, shy, and compliant twin. I would act out in some very unhealthy ways, such as compulsive overeating, drinking, and spending money like it was inexhaustible. My way of dealing with life situations within my twin-ship was very unhealthy and immature. Denial was a tool I used to help me feel protected – I thought maybe my problems would just go away, and this was a belief which I later learned kept me protected. I wanted to either deny that problems existed, or just avoid them all together by distracting myself with other activities. In addition, I would rationalize, pretend, and minimize the situation, lying to myself that I was making more out a situation than there was, or telling myself that my situation was not that bad. Over and over, I told myself not to be true to myself, after all, I didn't want to cause trouble or have anyone become upset with me. So again, denial was what was familiar to me.

"Everything is an opportunity, even if it doesn't seem like it."

I want to introduce you to a process which, as you follow these steps, will bring alignment into your life, with greater happiness, freedom, and love. I only ask that as you approach the steps in this process, you trade in judgement for curiosity, and trust the process – this means surrendering, and seeing these steps in the order they are presented, as they build upon the previous ones.

This first step in this process is a two-for-one, incorporating steps one and two that I mentioned earlier,

"Stepping Back" from your situation and "Letting Go" of obstacles and limiting beliefs that are keeping you stuck and may be holding you back from a better solution. This portion of your journey is about putting distance between you and your challenge, and it works, whether it is a current challenge, or something that has been a long-term problem due to repeated patterns of your childhood programming.

It may be unfamiliar and uncomfortable to open yourself to something new, and if this is you it may be helpful to ask yourself, "What do I have to lose and what do I have to gain?"

Up until that point, my life was certainly not ideal or truly what I wanted in my heart of hearts. The first time I let go, I was completely coming from a place of desperation, I was at the end of my rope, not seeing any choices available to me towards a working solution.

I asked myself, "What if I could change my experience and my outcomes to be more in alignment with who I want to be, and the outcomes I want?"

One of my "old beliefs" was that it was "selfish" to want something for myself. Boy did I need to have a "breakthrough" there! I had been programmed to be selfless which aided in how I felt… invisible, and it was as if what I wanted was not important. I believed I was not "good enough," and my self-esteem really took a hit with these "old beliefs." So, as I let go of these "old beliefs," I could be different without *remembering* to be different! This sounded like I did not have to take advice to have a new experience, and *wow*, I liked the sound of that! This seemed almost effortless to me in comparison to what I thought "change" meant. My definition of change was related to pain – excruciating emotional and mental pain – due to all my resistance. This was a huge differentiator in my experience to what I thought change was supposed to be like, and how it truly can be manifested and realized.

So, the first part, "Stepping Back," is about creating distance between you and your problem and programing. Again, your programming is what you were given at an early age of two or three, and this determined how you made decisions about yourself and the world, coming from your parents and caretakers. Therefore, the reason why it is important to step back and get distance between you and your programming is that the distance opens up the opportunity to see a situation from a new fresh perspective. This is priceless!

Why is it important to see a situation from a new perspective? What is the benefit of that?

Well, if you can see a challenge from a new perspective, you are likely to see and create more choice and possibility from a more positive space. This gives you the opportunity to step back from an emotional reactive state, based on your programming, and move you into an observer position. You can now be enabled to see with eyes of curiosity, love and compassion, rather than that old familiar place of fear, anger, stress and judgement – you know what I mean, that knee-jerk reaction which always seems to get away from you. So, with this new strategy, a new reality can be created with different choices which better serve you. You can now be in the present moment creating a new experience, and a better outcome going forward. The situation may not change quickly, or it may not change at all, but *you* will absolutely change! You are, in essence, saying, "I *choose* an experience of surplus rather than an experience of depletion, even if others don't!" This is *empowering*!

Transformation is a continual process of letting go!

Indeed, the core of transformation is a continual process of letting go. You've probably heard the saying, "happiness is an inside job." This concept is about giving you a way to collapse and release your "old story," and help you to recognize patterns of victimization, how you are creating negative energy and experiences, and uncovering obstacles that keep you stuck – basically, it may be the right time to let go of your "younger twin." Remember, your programming that I talked about earlier? It is a way to let go of your "old beliefs," "old ideas," and "patterns of being," and create new ones.

Remember, I mentioned earlier about "being different" without having to "remember to be different." In my practice, I use a method called Transformational Coaching Method (TCM©). TCM© has to do with rewiring neural patterns, changing the reaction of thought patterns in the brain. It opens up new pathways in the brain so patterns become automatic, and do not require will power or discipline to remember to be different – you are just different! This is a little of the science behind this method.

This concept of "Letting Go" was completely foreign to me. My limiting beliefs went something like this: *try harder, do better, be perfect.* If something wasn't working, it would work or work even better or faster if I tried harder. This thought process made sense to me. Remember, fear and anger were my constant companions – this was the way I had survived until I truly began to live. I was driven, and I expected others to be too. I believed that controlling, worrying, caretaking, and forcing solutions was the way I showed that I cared, and I believed this would positively affect the outcome I desired. Even when I felt entitled to "be right" when I was right, it was not working. This was my programming. Eventually, I found I could be right without *having* to be right, if you get my drift. I knew I had transformed!

These messages are tricks people play on you. No matter how hard you try, you think you
have to do better. Perfection is elusive and keeps you stuck and unhappy. It is an unattainable goal, and one that sets you up for failure. Perfection gives you no space to feel good about what you've done and accomplished, because it is never good enough. Until these obstacles are uncovered, and your brain is rewired with a different message, you will never feel good enough, or be good enough, as you are.

Relationships are challenging, but the twin-ship has its own core issues that may have been the result of expectations, misconceptions, or comparisons, which have a definitive impact on self-worth, as I talked about in an earlier chapter. Because of these ways of thinking and being, twin relationships can be difficult, and navigating through all this can be especially tricky. You may be thinking, "What do I let go, and what do I preserve?"

By shifting to a new perspective, letting go of old limiting beliefs, imposed behaviors, and your programming, you will gain clarity in your thinking and directness in your own choices. You will have a clearer definition of yourself and it will open the way to healing and having a more peaceful relationship with yourself, and possibly with your twin. You will understand that if you want something from your twin, but cannot get it, it is perfectly okay. This may not be a possibility now, but it may be a possibility later. You will not have to give up who you are and what you want when being a people pleaser, but you will be empowered to make healthy and appropriate choices about where and how to get what you want. You will begin to let go all those expectations, misconceptions, limiting beliefs, and will form a new relationship with yourself (and your twin).

Through my own experience, I have found a new courage and strength in the concept of "Stepping Back and Letting Go." I have opened to the nearness of a Spirit of Love, – or Creative Intelligence or Life Force, however you identify – and when I do this following exercise, what I like to call "magic," something beautiful happens. As you let go and let Spirit Love, you are opening a new space and co-creating with Source for a shift. New ways of thinking and being for yourself will occur, and you will have love, new opportunities, and new ways of being. Like birds in flight who give up their wings to the flow of air, you too can trust and lean into the currents of Spirit Love which carry you to your destination and heart's desires.

The following questions will help you to draw upon your curious side and help you to gather as much insight into yourself as you begin the process of "Stepping Back and Letting Go!"

- What is the one thing you can celebrate in your life right now?
- What do you want *more* of in your life?
- What do you want *less* of in your life?
- Where do you feel certain and uncertain in your life?
- What are the top three most important things in your life?
- What needs to change?
- What are some common challenges/patterns you see showing up over and over again?
- What is in conflict or not in alignment?
- Are you ready for this to be different?

- What's the breakthrough you want to create around this?
- Where do you feel the strongest sense of love and connection right now?
- Where, if at all, do want more love and connection in your life?

"I was holding on to everything I thought I needed, but everything I needed was available and given to me when I let go."

Making peace with yourself and your past, whatever your philosophy or beliefs are, can allow us to find some common ground. Our past was neither an accident nor a mistake. You have been who you needed to be with the necessary people. You can embrace your past with all its history, pain, imperfections, mistakes and maybe even tragedies. Whatever your past has been, it is uniquely yours; it was intended for you, exactly as it was.

I will add to that, saying that I believe there are no coincidences –you are reading this book because you were called here, to this place, right here, and right now.

Chapter 5
Exploring and Connecting with Spirituality -
Religion vs. Spirituality

"Every moment, feeling, and experience is perfectly orchestrated
for your destiny. Nothing happens to you; everything
happens for you."

I think it is important for me to provide you with some personal background/history to my experience with religion versus spirituality as you can begin to explore your experience and belief system. Remember, I am relating my experience, and I am not here to judge anyone's experience. I'm just here sharing mine.

As a child, I was raised in New Jersey, my twin and I were in the birth order of middle having an older and younger brother. In my upbringing… my understanding of my childhood religion was there are 10 Commandments which I viewed as rules, saying "do this," and "don't do that." If I broke any of these rules, there was the possibility

I would burn in hell for all eternity. There was a distinction made between "mortal" and "venial" sins. The big, grave sins were unforgiveable – these were, I believe, the seven deadly sins, and they were the ones to stay away from like murder, adultery, and stealing. The rest of the sins fell into the category of the venial sins, such as hurting someone, and selfishness. These seemed to be in the realm of just being human – having faults, bad habits, but striving to be better each day.

Then there was the formidable confessional box. I remember it being dark and scary, with a screen separating me, the sinner from the priest. I couldn't see the priest, and I'm not sure whether or not he could see me, but I assumed he could not. I felt so much fear, guilt, and shame having to do this weekly. After confession came the penance, which usually consisted of something scripted and routine, the same prayers to say over and over. The effect this experience was having on me was that I was slipping away from being honest, in favor of just doing what was expected of me. It became so routine and I was running out of things to say.

Now, if you considered yourself good at practicing your religion, and wanted to follow the rules because you did not want to burn in hell for all eternity, but you were running out of things to say in that dark box, you might have done what I did – start getting creative and begin lying in the confessional. I thought if I kept repeating the same sins over and over each week, the priest would think I was lying, so I started making my confession up, I started lying right there to the priest – sounds pretty crazy, huh? Eventually, I completely fell away from these absurd behaviors, and I became a rebellious teenage, no improvement here. Religion was very stifling, and it was cramping my style. I started to break all the rules, including not dressing the same as my twin. I was beginning to notice I was not my twin – we did not have the same taste in clothes. While she seemed more conservative in her own style, I was flashier without going overboard. I just liked more bling!

I continued to go to the church of my childhood where I was taught *about* God, but I was not taught to *experience* God. That job was left for the priests alone. Back in the day, the mass was said in Latin and the priests would tell us the message in English. Religion gave me a set of rules that I could not seem to follow, while I constantly felt that I was falling short, helping me load up the guilt. I was trying to be following my religion and yet feeling so much fear, guilt, and shame. Something was really wrong with this picture for me.

Learning about God and experiencing God is very different. It is the difference between Religion and Spirituality. Religion was stagnant, like the Dead Sea, while Spirituality was about relationship – it was flow, movement, connection, and communication. Religion provided no connection to a Power Greater than, while Spirituality opened the space for choice in the matter. I was quite intrigued by this, and I wanted to know more. My own journey into Spirit has evolved into having a life that I could not even imagine was possible. On my own, however, it was impossible.

The difference came for me when the life I was living felt so empty that I had very little meaning and purpose. I wondered how other people seemed to be happy, successful, and fulfilled. There was definitely a dimension to my life that was missing.

Before we begin to explore fulfillment, we need to uncover what is blocking this path for you and what is required by this path of you.

I would like this experience to be in flow for you, as it is for me, so let's begin with a meditation that I wrote:

You can begin by taking a few deep, cleansing breaths,
feeling grounded and centered.

*Your feet have been set on a path, a path
which was designed just for you. It is firm,
supportive, guiding, and full of ease and
flow, light and love. As you walk, you notice
a sign at the edge of this path, and as you
get closer, you see words, words of
affirmation – it says, "This is the way to
truth, walk in it." You begin to smile, and
your feet feel more secure on the path
because you know it is just for you. Notice
how you feel as you walk – carefree, light,
happy? Notice how your body feels –
energetic, carefree and amazed? You may
feel like skipping like a child.*

*You may notice as you walk, is the path
smooth? Are there obstacles, ups and
downs? You sense there is a power in you
and around you, guiding and protecting you
as you take each step. There is no place for
worry or doubt on your path, you are
perfectly supported wherever you walk.*

Now, as you are crossing a bridge to the other side, you see yourself already there. But something is different. You seem different – you are totally alive; you are happy and healthy in every way. You are motivated to keep walking this path because you connected and have found yourself again. And what joy this brings to you! You discovered many gifts which bless and enrich you and bring you all the things you have desired for so long. They are now brought forth to be manifest in your life in a way you could not believe was possible for you – being, and connecting, and finding your own autonomy and individualism, apart from your twin, while still having your twin.

These obstacles, that once pulled you in every un-serving direction, no longer have power or influence over you. They have fallen away as you have chosen one choice after another, aligning with your truest, best version of yourself.

Cyndi Rutherford (CHC)

"To find fulfillment is to dream, to strive and struggle, and often times, to engage with adversity."
– Anna Rowley, Ph.D.

It is important to remember that life's wisdom comes through the ups and downs as you take time for reflection. This is vital to your spiritual path, as is examining your own belief system. Ask yourself:

- Is your current belief system working for you?
- Is your belief system based on fear, guilt or shame or faith, trust and intuition?
- What is your life like when you are not connected?
- What is your life like when you are connected?
- How do you identify that Power which is greater than you?
- What shifts in your life when you are deeply connected?
- Is your belief system connected to unhealthy dependencies?

Switching from Co-Dependency to God-Dependency

In my experience being the younger twin, I was passive and compliant, while my twin was dominant and more independent. I overly identified with her and became enmeshed with her because I was not taught healthy boundaries, so boundaries became blurred. I could not be possible to have my own identity because I had no sense of self. I wanted and expected my twin to take care of me and make me feel whole – I was always looking for a mother figure, since my own mother was not present due to her illness. As twins, we were set up to believe that we had the same identity. Anything that opposed this idea was considered to be a threat to the twin relationship. Enmeshed twins have very little capacity to focus solely on themselves because they do not view themselves as having autonomy. They have little capacity to develop apart from the twin-ship for fear they would alienate their twin, and so, most choice is based on need, not want.

A healthy closeness would mean having separate and authentic lives, and it would reflect two distinct individuals having a strong sense of self, while still having time together and enjoying each other's company. This relationship would be based on choice, not neediness.

When the family structure is healthy and children have a strong attachment to the parents, the result is opportunity for each twin to have space to identify who they are, and to feel supported and loved as the individuals they are.

If this is not the case, the adult twins can recognize that co-dependency exists and make a commitment to themselves to grow as individuals, having a distinct sense of self, and can now embrace a healed twin-ship that becomes loving and caring instead of needy and insecure. After that, it is more likely the twin-ship becomes flexible and resilient and will no longer create feelings of resentment, aloneness, and abandonment.

Patterns and Characteristics of Co-Dependence

The following is just a small checklist I offer you as a tool to help identify these traits as you begin to understand co-dependency:

Denial Patterns

- Demanding their needs be met by others
- Having difficulty identifying feelings
- Denying, minimizing, altering how they really feel
- Thinking they can take care of themselves without any help from others

Low Self-Esteem Patterns

- Having difficulty making decisions
- Having difficulty admitting mistakes
- Judging what they think harshly, as if it is never good enough
- Looking to others to provide their sense of safety

Compliance Patterns

- Extremely loyal, remaining in harmful situations for too long
- Compromising their own values and integrity to avoid rejection or anger
- Afraid to express their feelings, beliefs, or opinions when they differ from others
- Giving up their truth to gain the approval of others; often compromising and overly accommodating

Control Patterns (Or, Co-Dependents Often…)

- Believing people are incapable of taking care of themselves
- Attempting to convince others what to do, think, or feel
- Freely offer advice and direction without being asked
- Becoming resentful when others decline their help or reject their advice

Avoidance Patterns

- Avoiding emotional, physical, or sexual intimacy as a way to maintain distance
- Push-and-pull pattern
- Allowing addictions to people, places and things to distract them from intimacy in relationships
- Refusing to give up their self-will to avoid surrendering to a Power Greater than themselves

So how does one switch from a life of dependence on others for their emotional well-being to a spiritual life based on a Power Greater than for their emotional well-being? How does one fill in that gap? It is called *faith* – faith and belief that this power supports you and has your back, as a best friend would. Growing spiritually is a process. It can start really small, with just an opening to the possibility that there is a higher power, and it can evolve into believing in this power – having a faith that works in good times and bad times. It will require you to trust and to let go on a level you've not understood yet, much like a child trusting a loved one. Whenever called upon, this power will be there. There is a wonderful, amazing essence to this Power….. love, peace, power, and God is constant, comforting and jealous.

Yes, that's right! This power wants to be first in your life. This power wants your happiness, but you have to want it too. Together you can co-create a life that you truly want, beyond anything you can dream or imagine.

Remember, though, we are spiritual beings trying to have a human experience.

Chapter 6
Finding Forgiveness

"The most efficient states for change are curiosity and amazement, not judgement."

I can't speak about another's guilt; I can only speak about mine. Being co-dependent and a people-pleaser meant that I was afraid you would abandon me, and I would have no identity. I over identified with my twin, and for years I had no sense of self apart from her. Being raised in an environment of alcoholism and co-dependency, I had a lot of issues; perfection, guilt, oversensitivity, anger, and fear followed me wherever I went, and wreaked havoc in all my relationships. A long time ago, a friend of mine told me that I had a well of guilt so deep she couldn't see the bottom. My family and religious background produced this fear and guilt.

As I matured in my awareness of having certain limitations as a human being, and yet having unlimited possibilities with God as my source of life, I came to see that my "well of guilt" was so very deep, and that just maybe I needed a Power Greater than myself to help me.

This is my desire for you: to be open to having God's best for you. Realizing that my love is conditional and limited, but God's love is unconditional and full of unlimited possibility, I wanted to experience the unlimited power of God's forgiveness. This would sustain me and remove my guilt on a supernatural, spiritual plane, not just in the natural plane. This is a process, and "progress not perfection," is one of my favorite slogans.

Connecting with Yourself and Your Pain

The first stage of forgiveness is to identify who caused your pain by their actions or omissions. Begin to write a list of your offenders, even if they had no ill intent, and even if the person(s) are deceased. You can write these people a letter or speak to them, whichever way you prefer. Write their names and the situations which caused you emotional pain. Place yourself on the very top of the list, and write all the situations which come to mind that you have felt disappointed either in yourself or another, and record your feelings of guilt, shame, betrayal, abandonment, sadness, anger, fear, and isolation. Be as thorough as you can as you write, because thoroughness will have its own reward. This is *your* time now to let your feelings come. Whether your feelings gently rise to the top, come like a flood, or require you to dig for them like gold does not matter, because they truly are golden nuggets filled with light and healing.

As you are laying all of this out, tell it from the perspective of still being the victim, following the "old story" paradigm.

For example, write: because of how you treated me, or are still treating me, I feel (fill in the blank).

This is how you begin to get connected with your feelings. It is really important for your healing process to allow all your feelings – which have been buried, stymied, ignored, and minimized– the space for love and healing. It may be a beneficial for you to have good support during this part of the process.

You can trade judgement for curiosity, just notice what it is you are feeling, and this will begin to give you clarity on your journey to forgiveness. Love yourself for having these feelings, and remember feelings are neither right nor wrong – there is no judgement, your feelings are yours. You will want to take a quiet, objective view. As you are recognizing, owning, validating and accepting your feelings, you now have the choice to let them go, as you did not give yourself this choice when you were stuffing, rationalizing, and minimizing your feelings.

It is vitally important to your healing to now embrace all your feelings – the good, bad, and ugly. By owning all of your feelings without judgement, your feelings will feel safe to come out and feeling them is the way you will move forward.

Just a thought, I want to interject here: owning and taking responsibility will begin to shift you away from blaming others and playing the victim. Remember, "We are always winning the game we are playing."

Feelings which are suppressed manifest in negative energy being stored within your body. This unhealthy practice impacts sleep, weight, mood, relationships, and your overall health.

There are options to start this process toward forgiveness. You can either tell it in story form, or you can simply make a list of the people with whom you were upset, or whom you may currently be upset with. It is whichever resonates with what is most true for you.

If you choose to write your feelings in story form, be sure you write about the person in third person. Here is another example of what I mean: my twin, Anne, hardly ever calls me. If we talk, I am always the one who initiates the call. I am feeling ignored and abandoned. I am feeling that I am not as important to her as she is to me. This makes me feel like I am not good enough.

You are now moving away from an unhealthy pattern of being to a healthy pattern of being, without the blocks of hard energy, and into more ease and flow. This represents your first step toward liberation from being a victim to an overcomer. You will experience a shift in your thinking and being. When we give other people the power to hold us in a sort of emotional bondage or control, we give our power away, and put ourselves in the position of feeling disempowered and victimized again. This is a way of withholding love, safety, and belonging. When I am feeling either disconnected from myself or others, it all begins with me. For example, if I desire something or someone to change and I am trying to force a solution, I am in a deficit. The outcome will be a negative feeling state, such as feeling ignored or disappointed. When I am judging that person, place, or thing to my expectation, this will probably create resistance and I will not experience my desire. However, when a person, place or thing is accepted with love as being exactly the way it is supposed to be at that moment, change can occur. It's paradoxical, like magic!

Hang in there with me for a little while, you're doing great! You are on your way to having the "old story" collapse. In Chapter 2 we were identifying your "faulty foundation" and collapsing the "old story." Well, here it is!

Go back to your story or your list – however the universe planned this for you and write out all the ways you were withholding love and holding judgement towards yourself and others, and wanting them to change. The purpose of this part of the chapter is to separate "facts" from "fiction." We are "meaning-maker machines." What I mean by this is that we attach meanings to our experiences so it makes sense to us.

We all have "strategies" for creating love, safety and belonging. These strategies got "coded" as a young child before the age of three. This is where we make important and significant choices about ourselves and our world for keeping love, safety, and belonging intact. What is really interesting as adults is that we continue to seek the same experiences as we replay the original strategy sequence.

I'm going to really slow it down here and we will take this frame by frame.

Frame 1: You are two-years-old. You're happy, with no worries, and everything is groovy baby!

Frame 2: A problem occurs. There is a break in love. You want to play with your twin, but she has a different idea. A sound is catching her attention from the other room, and full of curiosity, she runs to see where the sound is coming from. For a two-year-old, life is either awesome or bad.

Frame 3: A decision was made about you, your twin, and the world around you. This occurs in the part of your brain called the cortex, where information, sensory, and motor processing occurs, and it is trying to figure out why that bad thing just occurred! Why that break in love? You wanted to play with your twin, but she suddenly had a different idea and ran in a different direction. The one thing that is the most intolerable for a child is confusion – things failing to make sense.

In this way, we attach meanings to experiences, and we can't stand it when something doesn't jive. I used to try to make sense of it by putting meaning to it. I thought something was wrong with my dominant twin, or that something was wrong with my world, or that something was wrong with me – here comes the "I'm not loveable, I'm not good enough" programming.

The only survivable conclusion to draw here was that something was wrong with me, because if something was wrong with my twin, I would just die! Something being wrong with the world was also untenable to me, so the only way for that scenario to make sense was to decide something was wrong with me. This is how false, limiting beliefs are introduced into the psyche. Basically, this entire sequence was coded in the brain as necessary for my survival. Since we didn't die the first time I experienced this, my brain believed that this was the formula for staying alive. Interesting……

So how does this play out for adults? In order for you to be loved, you need to find someone who is going to run in the other direction when you want that fun, and you keep proving to yourself that there is something wrong with you. Here's the thing about beliefs, since they were coded into your brain around two or three-years-old, they aren't often accessible directly through language. You can't talk yourself out of it, because you did not talk yourself into it.

What is the fix for this? The brain needs to be rewired to think something positive. In my practice, my approach is to create good feelings, and then point you in the direction of your desired state. The first step in this is to build choice. Anyone can learn to create positive feelings and learn to behave differently to some degree or another. If we have a problem and only one choice, we feel kind of stuck. If we have two choices, we can choose between the two and this feels better. But if we have three or more choices, the situation starts to feel more freeing, as we have choice rather than "stuckness."

As I mentioned earlier, part of collapsing the "old story" is identifying these limiting beliefs. Check this list and see which belief you have the strongest feelings toward.

- I'm not good enough
- I'm not worthy of having love
- People always leave me
- I don't deserve to be happy
- I'm not loveable
- It's not safe to be me
- I'm always left out
- I am invisible
- Life is not fair
- Something bad will happen if I'm happy or successful
- No matter how hard I try, I can't have what I want
- Everyone is more important to me
- I don't deserve to be happy and successful

Reframing the Picture

Everything has a purpose and balance – nothing is wasted in the economy of the universe. There was a reason you formed those beliefs! Do you feel like the only purpose was to cause you suffering? Well, these beliefs certainly did bring you pain. However, what if something else was true? What if your soul chose these experiences for you? What if they were hand-picked, just for you, so you could begin to get unstuck from the "old story" and co-create with a Power Greater than yourself, a power of your own understanding?

Most of all, be gentle with yourself. These old ideas and limiting beliefs have been a part of your operating system for a long time. Don't be critical or beat yourself up for not letting go of them sooner. Don't be angry or upset with yourself when you realize that you have created your life based on a state of false beliefs. Welcome to the human race! This is what we do; it is how we are wired. Remember, you're always creating something. You are either creating unlimited possibility, a successful, flowing life, or a life based on negativity, lack and stuckness. You may be stuck in limiting possibility, but you are always creating.

On a daily basis, practicing gratitude for experiencing an awakening to the truth of the matter will continue to advance your journey.

And remember, *staying stuck is a choice*!

Chapter 7
Create Your Self-Portrait

"I choose an experience of surplus instead of an experience
of depletion, even if others don't."

My purpose for creating this chapter for you, my reader, is for you to be inspired and feel empowered as you begin to create a portrait of yourself as an individual, and to have your own independent life. I want you to give yourself permission to be *bold* and *honest*, and for you to be true to yourself by finding your own identity, being an individual, having your own voice and truth, and for you to grow into yourself with grace, purpose, ease, and flow. I want you to understand that together we will create a safe space to love and fully express yourself without any fear of consequences. Go ahead and make a declaration to yourself: *I have a birthright to be myself, and I will emerge from this process a truer version of myself.* Say, "yes," to yourself!

There, you spoke it, loud and proud. Enter into this chapter with determination that you will not entertain fear, which, by the way, stands for "False Evidence Appearing

Real," because fear will try to hinder you, just as self-doubt will. Fear of losing my twin and fear of losing myself kept me in a state of being stuck. Make a promise to yourself that if fear and self-doubt should show up – which they will – you can journal about them and ask them, "What gift are you wanting to give to me?" In the quietness and stillness, listen to your inner voice, because you have more wisdom inside you than you realize. You can tap into this source with curiosity – the most efficient states for change are curiosity and amazement, not judgement.

I really wish I'd had a road map to creating my own identity apart from my twin, because it was a very messy process. I learned that life is messy – we are human beings and we make messes. I started to forge a path, and it took years, and I did not have to know the 'how" of it, I just had to make a beginning, because as I mentioned in the first chapter, I had a "breakdown before the breakthrough." It was the most intense and difficult change in my life to have to walk through. However, as I began to move forward, I began to get in touch with what I truly wanted.

I really wanted to have a more stable life as this was a dream come true for me. I wanted to stop being afraid of finding out who I was because I was also afraid that I would not like her. I wanted to give myself permission to go on a journey of discovering that it is okay to want to have a life of my own and most of all it was okay to be me. I asked myself, "What are your own desires?" "What are your core values?" "What is it that matters the most to you?" "How do you want to make a difference in the world?" How would making these choices affect the dynamics of my relationship with my twin?"

So, what you will be creating for yourself is an identity, separate from your twin, that feels right for you and aligns with the truest highest version of yourself. This is not the time to hold back. I dare you to get a little "wild and crazy!" You have permission to color outside the lines – anything goes, so trust yourself, it will be alright. This is not a once-over, it is just the beginning of a process into discovering who you are. Are you excited? I am so grateful to have you on this journey into discovery, because when I started, I thought I was the only twin who felt as I did. I carried shame inside me that I was not even aware of. I was still under the illusion and "false belief" that the best of twins didn't fight and argue the way we did. As I was doing my research for writing this book, this journey became a healing process for me, as I was able to let go of the shame I'd been carrying when truth entered my life and I could let go of that false belief.

Let's look back on your journey to finding your own identity. In the first step, you connected with the concept of "Stepping Back and Letting Go," where you began to identify with having a clear perspective regarding what it is that you want to change, what areas are shaky, and what is the one thing you want to work on , which would make the biggest difference in your life.

The next step in this process for creating a "Portrait of Yourself" is to establish a well-formed outcome. There are five criteria for meeting your desired state.

A well-formed outcome is:

- Stated in the positive: it says what you want, not what you don't want.

- Initiated and maintained by yourself: you don't need to rely on someone else changing (i.e. your twin)

- It is achievable with the time frame you give to it

- It has a specific sensory-based description, so you know how it feels or looks – it would be easy to measure, or we have a description that would tell us when we have it

- It is an appropriate size – the biggest chunk to be worthwhile, yet small enough to feel/be attainable

Without a clearly defined outcome, creating a "portrait" is difficult, because, if you are like me, you lose focus. Instead, you should track your progress and understand key pieces which need to be addressed to reach just 1% of growth each day, week, or month. Just keep telling yourself, "small hinges swing big doors."

The following is an exercise you can do which will support you in having a deeper sense of embracing your desired outcome, and can bring the awareness of what you want into view. As yourself:

- What do I want for myself in terms of my relationship with my twin?
- What would it look and feel like to have balance in my twin-ship?
- What challenges or difficulties would I need to overcome in order to get there?
- In order to have my own identity, what would I need to let go of?
- What have I been tolerating/putting up with that is no longer serving me?

- Who might benefit in my life if I make these
  changes?
- Who else might be impacted positively or
  negatively?
- What would it look like if the situation were
  resolved?
- Does that feel like the truth?
- What am I thinking about myself that makes this
  vision of myself possible?
- What becomes possible for me from this place
  of possibility?
- If I am able to give your present self any words
  of wisdom for the journey ahead, what might
  they be?
- What would having healthy boundaries look
  like?
- What would it feel like to have my own voice,
  to have my own truth?
- What would the experience of attaining some of
  my goals be like? How would stepping into that
  feel? How would claiming yourself and your
  power impact my life?
- What would I have to believe in order to have
  that experience?

- If I were to embrace my own life, while still preserving my twin-ship, who, if anyone, am I worried about losing a sense of belonging with?

The Two States of the Mind and Body

"Every moment, feeling, and experience is perfectly orchestrated for your evolution. Nothing happens to you – everything happens for you."

Survival

- Stress
- Contraction
- Dis-ease
- Imbalance
- Breakdown
- Closed-mindedness
- Separation
- Fear/Anger/Suspicion

Creation

- Relaxation
- Expansion
- Contentment
- Congruence
- Breakthrough
- Open-mindedness
- Connectedness
- Love/Joy/Trust

My breakthrough came after breaking my addiction to drugs and alcohol, and it only came as a result of an emotional breakdown, as I've previously mentioned. It was *difficult*! The faulty foundation, or programming, in which I stood was collapsing under my feet. YAY!! I realized I was suspended in a complete place of unknowing and uncertainty. All the "old ideas" were gone – all the answers I thought I had were *gone*! I felt completely untethered. I thought I had life figured out, but I was wrong! I couldn't go back, and I couldn't move forward. I contemplated suicide daily. I was *stuck* like I've never been stuck before. This experience was really different.

Before, I could always pull out one of my survival tools to squeak through, but I could not do that this time! It was a time of complete deflation and defeat. I was surrendering the faulty foundation. *Finally*, I had a choice now, which I was not ready to have earlier, and one I had never used in earnest, as I did after my breakthrough.

I asked for help. This had always been hard for me, because my programming said to "pull yourself up by your bootstraps," and both God and others had always disappointed me. I could not trust anyone, which is how I came to rely on myself. None of this seemed to be working for me, and I asked for help because I realized my identity crisis was tripled with addiction and co-dependency, and was completely beyond me. I felt completely powerless to do anything about my problem by myself.

I turned to a Power Greater than me, and together I call this power G.O.D., which stands for "Good Orderly Direction" in my mind. After all, what did I have to lose? I checked in with this power I didn't know. From many setbacks and failures, I came to realize self-reliance is not always the best course of action. I also realized that failure is only feedback. This reframe was priceless. It meant I did not need to suffer with failure as I did in the past, and I learned suffering is optional. It's really odd, how, as human beings, we resist the very thing which will be the needle-mover in our lives.

The pain is not necessarily in the changing – the pain is embodied in the resistance to it, and life has a way of persistently knocking until we answer the call. I was 33 when I had my breakdown and became suicidal. In order for me to stay alive – I had three children all under the age of ten, by the way –life was calling on me to change everything: my thinking, my relationship with a Power Greater, with myself, with my twin, my husband, and my children. All of my relationships were impacted.

There were some people who were not happy with me, because I was emerging from this experience different. I was no longer a doormat and victim, and I had the courage to stand up for who I was. I needed to come to terms with the fact that my twin had her own understanding and opinion of my circumstance. It was a "hot topic" for us, so we avoided talking about it. We were not raised in a healthy environment with healthy communication skills. At that time in my life, I believe a separation was in motion. Space was created for me to start on the journey to find my own identity apart from my twin. I realized that if I did not break free from my unhealthy dependency on my twin, I would never be an independent person with my own autonomy. I believe as I shed the "old story" and the "old me" I was becoming a stronger, confident, more capable woman which my twin never really understood. I was met with disapproval and misunderstanding, and this is completely understandable. I was always looking for my twin's approval and never getting it; putting her first. I needed to learn a lesson. It was not her approval I needed it was mine. During this process I realized I had a choice to make. I could go back to the familiar and be unhappy or I can keep moving forward knowing I would risk losing my twin. This was so difficult! Why did it need to be this way?

I needed to let go, take a risk resulting in having my own self and being happy today. There was a part of me whispering, 'this is not God's best for you,' and I healed from my past and I no longer live in that self-imposed misery. This is how I was inspired to write "BECOMING UN-TWINED." By taking the right steps which I have laid out in these chapters, I am free today. As I wrote and reflected on my own journey, I was healed of shame about the twin mystique….'twins are close and they never fight'. This is just not true! I kept this a secret for years until I was faced with the truth and dropped this belief like a hot rock. I wanted to be a part of the solution by being transparent enough to make a difference for other twins who identified with the same struggle to be free to love themselves enough to embrace the possibility of having a new life. It was the beginning of self-acceptance, love, and giving myself permission to find my independence, and I learned my happiness was not dependent on my twin. I had a CHOICE. This was really unfair for me to expect her to do this job for me. There is always a positive intention in the situation, and this was it!

If you have formed a strong attachment with your twin – which is certainly the norm for twins – remember that being dependent on your twin for love, and a sense safety and belonging will not give you a chance to form a secure sense of self. On some level, you may feel the need to separate for a time so you can have space for reflection and an opportunity to make your own decisions to mature and grow. On the other hand, you may create scenarios to create distance through fighting with your twin and becoming irritated for no reason. There may be misunderstanding when one twin grows in a different direction than the other, creating feelings of disloyalty to the twin-ship.

Sometimes, when programming has been so damaging in childhood, some twin-ships can become toxic and you may need more space to heal through these issues. It is really important to recognize unhealthy ways of getting distance from your twin, in order to maintain your own individuality and autonomy. It is important to acquire a posture for tolerating differences in the relationship and forming a loving acceptance for your twin, in order to preserve the relationship and move in a healthier direction together. Every person wants to experience their own individuality, and it is doubly important in a twin-ship for this to happen.

Too much togetherness will actually stifle the relationship, as will too much separation. It is vital to the life of the relationship to be in balance, and if your relationship is out of balance, you won't have the experience of being in a healthy twin-ship.

Chapter 8

Rise, Ignite Your Spark!

"Desire is not selfish, it is wise. It's a compass pointing you in the direction of your life's purpose."

If you are still reading and hanging out with me, you are doing *awesome*!

Have you realized it yet that someone gave you a script to follow for your life? It could have been your parents, primary caregivers, or teachers, but there is nothing wrong with the script – it has worked for countless others. Have you tried really, really hard to follow this script, but in some areas of your life, you're still not getting the results you want? Does this resonate with you?

I have an example of following a script that comes to mind. I was in labor and delivery with my second child – I'd been through Lamaze classes twice. I was following the script and working really hard because I wanted to succeed, but the next thing I knew I was being prepped for a C-section. My brain was scrambling! "What do I do, what do I do?" I wondered. This is not what I want! This is risky, but I have to do something different! I did something so contrary to my beliefs! A voice quietly spoke to me, "Maybe you should stop working so hard at this 'labor.'" After all, it's a process, right? Millions of women have babies *and* this was not my first! I decided to stop trying to do it perfectly as with trying to control my breathing and following the script – in fact, I abandoned the script! For me, not being compliant was a scary risk, but I did not want to have a C-section, because I did not want my body to be cut open. I started to just go *with* the labor, and not worry about doing it perfectly, and I just relaxed as best I could. I found a natural flow to my labor. I was no longer forcing it, trying to change it, or trying to rush it. After all, who likes pain? I just wanted to get the labor finished! The next feeling I had was complete surprise and amazement. I was in the final stage of labor, and my course to C-section was completely changed. *Wow*! I realized there was a timing in the universe that is perfect. I believe this was the first time I was consciously aware of "trusting the process." This choice was a big needle-mover in my life – this was surrendering the control and trusting a different way, contrary to what I believed. My outcome became my desire.

Life is good! Life offers us choice-points! Depending on which choice is made, your decision can impact you for a day, a week, a year, or a decade.

Change is a matter of perspective – it can be viewed with resistance, or it can be embraced. When we have resistance to change, our energy becomes constricted and we may feel uptight or stressed. We put our heads down, buck the winds of change and just hope everything will go back to normal. The culprits behind this resistance are usually fear and self-doubt. They are blocks to having what you want, and they only keep you stuck. In Chapter 4 I talked about letting go of limiting beliefs and self-sabotage because these are fear-based, and as you continue to rely instead on power source, these fears will lose their hold. Our comfort zone, routines and status quo are all enemies to change, and that which keeps us stuck.

The easier way to approach change is with an attitude of openness, curiosity, and acceptance. Change is inevitable and desirable. We can trust ourselves and our intuition and it will never guide us in the wrong direction – it is totally reliable. Letting go and surrendering fear opens the pathway to change.

What would it be like to feel a greater sense of self, belonging, and a deeper connection to a Power Greater?

Ask yourself what it would feel like to embrace a greater sense of confidence and ease, because this can be possible for you.

Unlocking Your Personal Power

There is a creative intelligence within you. You've heard the expression, "trust your gut." Tapping into your "gut wisdom" is your natural intuition, and intuition is trusting what you already know to be true. We have been taught to not trust our gut and to outsource our intuition and doubt ourselves, but the truth is, we are the best expert when it comes to our own life.

When you begin to tune into yourself, you will find that you have so much wisdom to draw on, which comes from a Power Greater. You cannot always trust your feelings, but you can always trust your gut. However, when you choose to not trust your gut – because you've allowed fear to dominate – it sets you up for others to be in control, and you've given your personal power away. If you are really tuned in to this voice, you can trust it to give you wisdom for your life, and if you choose to not listen over time, the voice becomes distant and it becomes harder to maintain a connection with it.

Empowering Yourself

"You can think, you can make good decisions that are right for you, you can take care of yourself, and you can tune in to your intuitive, inner-wisdom."

Although we all make mistakes sometimes, we are not mistakes. It is okay to be imperfect. We can make a choice, and if it is not the right one, we can simply make another. Sometimes we learn from our own experience, and sometimes we learn from other's mistakes. Other times, we can just change our mind if we get new information we did not previously have.

You are finding out that you have the freedom to grow and move at your own pace. You have a birthright to discover who you uniquely are, and it's absolutely OK to be you apart from your twin without feeling guilty. You no longer need to feel responsible for other's choices, and this also means you are accountable and responsible for your choices. You can forgive yourself for not knowing, and you can live and let live. You can find new purpose and happiness being your own individual self while you use your imagination to have your dreams. Your dreams come true when you believe in yourself and walk towards your dream each day. You are free to embrace and enjoy the magic of your own mind, intellect, spirit and wisdom.

Affirming Yourself

"I love myself, I am good enough as I am, my life is good, what I want and need is coming to me, and I am grateful for my life today."

You can make choices that line up with your core values today, and you can look at yourself and honestly ask what have you been withholding from yourself, and what has been stopping or standing in the way of having what you like. Positive thinking does not mean everything is wonderful. Positive thinking is a result of having faith when life is not going according to plan; it means you are grounded into a Power Greater. If something doesn't work out, remember that the universe has your back – whatever you wanted was not meant for you, so you have the energy to let it go and still be happy. Whatever we give our energy to, we empower. There is magic in empowering the good, because that energy attracts more positive energy.

The way you can empower positive energy is through affirmations. Your choice is not whether to use affirmations, because you've been affirming thoughts and beliefs since you were two or three-years-old. The choice you have now is *what you want* to affirm. Part of the process of affirming is letting go of the negative thought patterns to open the space for change for something new to emerge.

Self-Care

Motivation comes from knowing your why. There are three parts to self-care: body, mind, and spirit. Just knowing that it is important to take care of yourself will never take you the distance. Trying to conjure up steam may last for a day, if you can even get started. Motivation and commitment begin by asking one simple question: what is important about this for you?

Let's say your answer is positive thinking for a higher vibration in your life, and you ask yourself that same question again for each successive answer until your reach your *why*! Keep digging below the surface until you reach your deepest *why*! To give yourself a clue, the reason is usually attached to your heart. I suggest you then anchor it into something which has meaning for you – something you see or hear every day. For example, if you say, "Positive thinking is important for my mood and improves my intimacy," your anchor can be your wedding ring, get the picture?

Starting with our motivation, the idea of giving ourselves what we want and need may be confusing at first. It may even feel selfish. I just want to say, feelings aren't always facts! And you know what, it is okay to get a little selfish at first. After spending years of taking care of others, making the effort to begin to take the focus off others and transfer this focus to your own care might be just what you need. Placing yourself first will be challenging because that old thinking will want to creep in and pull you back into minimizing your wants and needs.

Gratitude is a powerful tool for lifting your mood and making this decision from a happy place. Asking yourself questions like, "What do I need? What is true for me? How do I take care of myself when I am feeling overwhelmed and out of control? What are my 5 non-negotiables? What makes me feel crazy?" Staying open to your feelings keeps you connected to your emotional health. If you feel angry, it's okay. Do not judge yourself for any of your feelings, because they are *your* feelings. You can own them – they are a part of you.

Feelings rise and fall, so it's okay to feel and accept them. Unresolved anger leads to hardened resentment. We were created to feel. Feelings are a gift. The best guide you have for your own self-care is your own inner-wisdom. Take time to tune in each day.

Journaling is a great way to connect with yourself and your self-care. Self-care is not difficult – once you get the momentum, you will find that it feels more natural. The challenging part is trusting your guidance and having the courage to follow through on it. This is proof that you are serious about loving yourself.

Balance

We can't talk about self-care without talking about balance. When you begin to take care of yourself and figure out what it is that you want and need, this will give you a measuring stick for tolerance. In the past, you may have tolerated too much or too little. You may have compromised too many pieces of yourself, or you may have expected too much from others. Either extreme is not in balance. Finding balance may take time, and there will be times things may get back out of balance but having the right tools will bring you back to your desired state. You can trust your intuition to bring you to a balanced place of love, tolerance, reasonable expectation, giving, and understanding.

Creating the change you want to see happen is not an "outside job," and it doesn't mean geographically separating yourself from your twin. Change is an "inside job." Becoming an individual, separate from your twin, means having healthy boundaries and dropping the comparisons and competition, which feeds low self-esteem. When I was participating with these patterns, I would always come out feeling less than my twin. Appreciating yourself and your twin for your individual personality and character traits is the main ingredient to having a balanced and healthy twin-ship.

Claim yourself and claim your greatness! Finding the freedom to connect with yourself as a stand-alone twin adds an expansion and fuller dimension to your life, which you previously denied yourself. Finding your own competency will strengthen your capacity to be confident in who you are. By being present to yourself you will find new purpose and meaning, giving you opportunities that were once void, but now have a space for creation. This is beautiful!

Anticipate good things to flow into your life. You will not need to control, worry, or figure it out, just surrender to your Power Greater each day, trusting your inner wisdom to lead you. This is how the good you desire will present itself. Trust your power source along with gratitude for your healing, your twin-ship, your desired change, your direction, your abundance and provision, your creativity, and your energy. Whatever it is you need – love, success, happiness –it has already been planned for you. Your job is to just remove the obstacles that are in your way. Trust the feedback the universe is giving you; this is only the task the universe is capable of: giving! You will be brought to it or it will be brought to you. The Power Greater wants to give you the desires of your heart and wants to see you have happiness and joy.

"What lies behind us, and what lies before us are tiny matters compared to what lies within us."
– Ralph Waldo Emerson

Chapter 9
A Moment of Clarity

"You're Always Winning the Game You're Playing."

What do I mean when I say this?

The first time I heard this quote, it seemed simple enough to understand. I wanted what was best for me, but was I showing up in alignment with what I wanted? If I was thinking and behaving in ways which were not in alignment with what I wanted, I was winning the game that I *was* playing! This was not good! This was not God's best for me!

What does this mean for you? It means understanding that you truly have control of your relationship, health, time, spirituality, money, and career. This is vital to understand – don't let your problem define your future. You have everything you need to make the changes you want for a more fulfilling, intentional and purposed life.

The value of becoming your own stand-alone twin is that you will be letting go of limiting beliefs which held you in bondage along with your victim mentality. This mentality lets your problem define your identity, and you are not your problem. Relationships, health, spirituality, money, time, and a career just don't happen to you – you are not a victim of circumstances. Rather, your current situation could possibly be a representation of the "younger twin," or your limiting beliefs, misconceptions, comparisons, emotional baggage.

You must forge your own unique path, as your path relates to what is true for you. When making decisions, you must attune yourself to your wants and needs, as these will line up with your core values. Twins don't always see eye-to-eye, and even if you and your twin disagree, you can accept her just as she is and you can accept that you will have disagreements – agree to disagree! Allowing for each other's opinions gives room for greater flexibility within your relationship. Focusing on your history with your twin – and honestly identifying your issues such as co-dependency, caretaking, comparisons and competition – opens up room for self-reflection and examination of twin-related issues you may find are holding you back from healthier relationships and a more fulfilling life. Focusing on your own thoughts and feelings will help you to gain a better a sense of control in your life. On the other hand, if the issues with your twin are left unresolved, and if you remain so entwined that you still don't know yourself as an individual, you will unconsciously carry your unresolved issues as baggage into every area of your life.

If and when you have some conversations with your twin, it's crucial to come to these with an open mind and heart and to trade in judgement for curiosity – leave behind blaming and finger-pointing, and ditch the "I'm right, you're wrong" mentality. You can be right, without **having** to be right, if you catch my drift. This prevents your twin from getting defensive, because if you always need to be right, the probability of an argument is elevated, and your conversation will most likely have a negative outcome, building resentment in to your relationship.

Making these shifts, resolving these conflicts, and growing beyond your problem enables you to align more with your authentic self, and you will know a new freedom and happiness.

To achieve these results, let's begin by looking at the ways you may give up your power and sabotage yourself in these areas of your relationships, health, finances, time, and career:

- Conflict: we are afraid of conflict with our twin, spouse, loved ones, and parents so we practiced avoidance

- Responsibility: we are afraid of growing up; we will make mistakes; somehow, we will mess up, and we would rather someone else handle the decisions and take care of us, to save us from the responsibility of being independent

- Thought: we are afraid of what others will think of us, especially anyone who matters to us

- Trust: I did not follow through again; I could not make it work again; I cannot trust myself to do this

- Failure: what if I fail at this? I'll never be good enough

- Disempower/Displeasure: if I'm successful, I may make things worse for someone I love (sometimes this is conscious, sometimes it is under the surface)

Let's have a look at "old limiting beliefs" and the emotional undercurrent when it comes to happiness. If you "old belief" is, "People won't accept me or love me if I am really happy," your emotional undercurrent is filled with shame and secrecy, as you minimize your happiness so others are comfortable.

- Old Belief: "People won't accept me or love me if I am really happy"
- ❖ Emotional Undercurrent: shame and secrecy (you minimize your happiness, so others are comfortable)
- Old Belief: "I am not good enough"
- ❖ Emotional Undercurrent: guilt (you need to over-deliver, or overcompensate)
- Old Belief: "I am not special or significant"
- ❖ Emotional Undercurrent: visibility (you fear standing out and being noticed)
- Old Belief: "The other person getting what they want is more important than getting what I want for myself"
- ❖ Emotional Undercurrent: fear of rejection (you fear that an opportunity may be lost, or that you will be told no)

It's really important that we take a look at how fear can be a very formidable foe. I mentioned earlier that fear stands for, "False Evidence Appearing Real." Fear can stop many of us dead in our tracks, because it will really try to beat us back as we are ready to try something new or different.

When fear shows up in my life, I like to look at it and laugh in its face. I say, "I know you! If you're showing up, this must mean I am doing something right, because you're here!" This attitude keeps things light and in the flow. However, if you are new to dealing with fear, it can be quite formidable. When taking a step out of your comfort zone, fear can show up as fear of being too fragile, fear of failure, fear of success, fear of being humiliated, or fear of what others may think of you. We start to second guess our wisdom, or our next step becomes shrouded in self-doubt until we talk ourselves right out of participating in our own best interest and life.

You may tell yourself, "I failed before! Why would this be different? I can't do it, it's too hard."

Maybe you have tried to move forward in the past and it didn't work. I am not here to convince you of anything, I just want to encourage you not to let your past define you.

My wish for you is that you will experience a moment of real clarity, a defining moment in your life when you can say to yourself truthfully, "Nothing changes if nothing changes." This moment will help you say yes to empowering and loving yourself enough to take that step toward finding your own path of light and love engraved with your name. Everything can change for you by having the desire to want something more for your life and believing that all things are possible to hearts and minds that are open to this possibility is key.

By uncovering these limiting false beliefs, misconceptions and expectations which were imposed on you, you can be free – free to experience a breakthrough from reoccurring patterns of self-sabotage, the issues of your twin-ship, and codependency, freeing yourself to discover who you actually are apart from your twin, while being freed from conforming to who you should be according to someone else's agenda. This will result in more alignment, allowing you to live in your own truth. This will only continue to give you greater happiness, creativeness and vibrancy throughout your life.

After engaging with this read, you can either put it on the backburner or place it neatly on your bookshelf with your other self-help books, choosing to try to go through this process alone. Although you have the greatest intentions, no lasting change occurs.

Why is this? The advantages of working with someone through your issues is that real, lasting, sustainable growth happens when we are in community co-creating with someone who has been where you are. It's like having a personal trainer versus exercising on my own. I would never push myself to the limits I would get with a trainer, because I quit on myself way too soon. I tell myself, "It's way too hard!"

I would never give myself the "stretch" that a trainer would, and I'm really not that great at keeping myself accountable. I go soft, or I procrastinate. I figure that I will do it tomorrow, or that everything seems so much more important than investing in my *life*!

You know how that goes: tomorrow doesn't come, and "nothing changes."

On the other hand, having a coach who has been right where you are and who understands your struggle to find yourself and has come through to the other side is different! I won't let you quit on yourself! You matter! I will offer you the support, accountability, and stretch you need to make these advances in your personal growth. You will be given the tools and strategies, and you will gain tremendous insight into yourself as you learn to trust yourself and make changes on a deeper level. Remember, "Happiness is an inside job."

Here is a golden nugget of wisdom for you: the word "responsibility" means we all have the ability to choose how we respond. By awakening your *roar* and shifting your sense of self, you will move toward building your *dream*!

In order for change to be successful, it is important to have courage, because change is uncomfortable, and you need to be willing to be uncomfortable. the end result will be worth it.

Will you choose to feel the fear anyway and be your own best friend by stepping up for your own growth in becoming uniquely you?

Remember, "Nothing changes if nothing changes."

Chapter 10
Believe in Yourself, You Have What It Takes!

"'There is never a downside to taking responsibility for your own experience."

"Time takes time." This may sound trite, but it's true. As you are giving yourself time to digest and take in the process laid out for you in this book you may be curious about what is it that you want, and it's even possible you already know what you *don't* want. Knowing what you *don't* want is a great way to start figuring out what it is you *do* desire.

Stepping back and gaining a new perspective, clearing out and letting go of old ideas, limiting beliefs, and false identity, and beginning to redefine your life, takes time. If you've been stuck in a problem for a while and you've sought help, but you're not moving forward, you may be losing hope. When I was running out of my own options, I absolutely needed the right help. To achieve success, sometimes we need to slow down to speed up.

A new journey *always* begins with making a *decision*, and it will take courage and a leap of faith into the unknown. It will take being open to discovery, and it will take letting go of the "problem under the problem." You may not know what that problem is yet, but aren't you worthy of finding it? This problem is the one that has kept you stuck in your "false identity." Fear will masquerade itself with many different faces, and it will tell you, "you better not look." It will try to intimidate you and beat you back into submission. Support is needed for the strongest of us. Looking and discovering takes courage, honesty, and self-love in order to take a bold step – that first step in the direction of your dream come true.

"A journey of a thousand steps begins with one," and making that decision in stepping back and letting go means making a choice to follow through with the other steps of the process with your desired dream in mind.

You may have been settling in your life because you don't know what's possible for you. Perhaps you are not fully engaging, or maybe your thought and behavioral patterns keep you stuck. You may feel like you are living in a glass house, looking from the inside out, seeing life just passing you by. You may not think it is because you are perpetually busy, but no real change is taking place toward finding your true self and purpose. Looking through a different lens can give you the insight you need for a spark to be ignited and for you to emerge with a vibrancy for life that was always available to you, but which you were unaware of this possibility. You just don't know what you don't know.

This is a powerful process, and as you surrender you learn to trust your intuitive self, building a connection with these parts of yourself and with a Power Greater than. You will find it is your birthright to find and connect to your true self, to have and feel your feelings, thoughts, desires, self-expression, and creative flow. This is how transformation happens. It is an ongoing experience and adventure of letting go and discovering yourself. You will begin to experience shifts which could not previously budge, and blocks of energy will be released into co-creating your unique life as an individual. Breakthroughs happen when the pain of remaining stuck is greater than the risk of change. Let go and thank your inner "younger twin" for all she has helped you to survive. She holds much of the wisdom for your transformation.

Surrender is a paradox – you must surrender to win. This takes a leap of faith, courage and strength, discarding the idea of surrender being a weakness which has kept you stuck.

You have decided to go through this process of shifting blocks of energy and letting go and uncovering the "blind spots" which no longer serve you, and have been standing in the way of you emerging as the amazing person you are, apart from your twin. This process will give you a greater sense of clarity as to your choices in a greater alignment for your life. You will have a new way of being without having to remember to be different.

Understanding co-dependency issues and roles of twins as caretakers, being dominant or passive twins, and how these roles played out in my twin-ship was freeing for me. Understanding our programming helped me release shame, guilt, and fear, and I was able to heal and accept myself and my twin for who we are. Trading in "Co-Dependency for God-Dependency" will elevate and free your life in ways beyond what you can think or imagine.

"I was always holding onto people, and they were always leaving."
– Lili St. Crow

Ask, yourself, "Is it enough for me to just read this book? Will that give me the transformation I want?" Is it your decision to want to have an *experience* and be open to something *new* and to open the pathway to *shine,* and if it is I invite you to realize your dream to come true.

Personally, I did not want to settle for second best – I wanted God's best for me. I wanted my *destiny*! I remember growing up and hearing someone say, "You can't have your cake and it too."

What? That was the craziest statement I ever heard. I thank God that I had enough spunk in me to defy this silly logic. I was no longer going to accept the negative messages the world was handing out to whoever would settle for these *big, bold lies*! I believed there has to be something better – there has to be more to life than what these messages were telling me. I felt so unfulfilled and empty on the inside. My philosophy is simple: *Don't quit five minutes before your miracle! Your dream come true is on its way!*

I found out that there are plenty of dream-stealers out there. They look like they are happy for you, but on the inside, they are negative, and misery is their constant companion. These energy zapping people want you to keep them company in their misery. Trust your gut wisdom and surround yourself with people who truly want your happiness and love you. You are *deserving* of this!

I will leave you with this inspiring quote by Anne Lamott:

"Lighthouses don't go running all over an island looking for boats to save; they just stand there shining."

Contact info: fullyaligned@outlook.com
Cyndi Rutherford
Certified Health/Life Coach